The 10-Day Smoothie Challenge

Lose Weight, Feel Great, and Transform Your Life from the Inside Out

By Drew Canole

www.fitlife.tv

Published by Drew Canole
Copyright © 2014, Fitlife TV LLC

ISBN: 1503166341
ISBN-13: 978-1503166349

Table of Contents

Disclaimer 5

Introduction 6

PART I: INITIATION **9**

    Digestion, Elimination, and Cleansing 10

    The Importance of Mindset 15

    Preparing for the 10-Day Challenge: Get Psyched! 17

PART II: ACTIVATION **40**

    Days 1 – 10 41

PART III: LEGACY **52**

    A Lifetime of Health: Where to Go From Here 53

PART IV: RESOURCES **56**

    Recipes 57

Thank You... 73

Freebies from Fitlife 74

About the Author 75

Disclaimer

The techniques, strategies, and suggestions expressed here are intended to be used for educational purposes only. The author, Drew Canole, and the associated www.fitlife.tv are not rendering medical advice, nor diagnosing, prescribing, or treating any disease, condition, illness, or injury. It is imperative that before beginning any nutrition or exercise program you receive full medical clearance from a licensed physician. Drew Canole and Fitlife.tv claim no responsibility to any person or entity for any liability, loss, or damage caused or alleged to be caused directly or indirectly as a result of the use, application, or interpretation of the material presented here.

Introduction

Welcome to the first day of the rest of your vibrant, healthy life! My name is Drew Canole and I'd like to personally welcome you to the Fitlife family. Remember, we're in this together. There is a reason you've picked up this book. Maybe you have some stubborn weight you'd like to release. Maybe your head is foggy and you can't think straight at work. Maybe you're struggling with a lack of energy and motivation, making it hard to get through the day without resorting to caffeine or other stimulants. Whatever your reason, I want to assure you that you're in the right place!

Most of us have had a rocky beginning in the nutrition world and it's really no wonder with all the misinformation out there, not to mention the relentless advertising and the availability of unhealthy foods. As a result, we are among the most overweight nations despite having extensive access to healthy food, education, and medical infrastructure.

But maybe that's the problem. What we've been taught to believe about food, nutrition, and health from the established medical community is a far cry from what is *actually* healthy.

Maybe this book is your last resort. If that's the case, then I'm so glad you're here. My favorite people to help are those who have lost hope. Read this book, take the smoothie challenge, and I promise you a new future of greater health and vitality than you've ever experienced before.

I know these promises are nothing new. You have every right to be skeptical because there are a lot of fads and gimmicks out there that just don't work. I want you to hang in there with me, though. I can personally vouch for everything I say here because I've been in your shoes. Three years ago, I was twenty-five pounds overweight, 22% body fat, tired, and lost. I didn't have any clear direction for my life and lacked motivation. I really felt like I was going nowhere, and I had the body to show for it. Then one day, my friend Mark introduced me to juicing. I was totally skeptical at first but drank the green drink he made for me anyway.

And then it hit me. Within fifteen minutes, every cell in my body seemed to be buzzing with life. It was a high I'd never experienced before. All the enzymes, aminos, and phytonutrients in that juice made me feel invigorated and alive. It was incredible! And unlike other substances people use to feel awake, like caffeine, my high stayed with me throughout the day. No energy crashes! I felt happier and more productive. It was then that I decided to include juicing in my daily routine.

I started with one juice a day. I found I was craving less of the foods I was eating before. Soon I wondered what it would be like to have two juices a day. Pretty soon, I felt so good I decided to embark on a three-day juice-only cleanse. After that, my life changed. The juicing worked wonders on my insides. I was cleansed. When I reintroduced solid foods, I found I could digest and absorb everything better than I ever had before. I noticed immediate results in my body composition, dropping down to less than 7% body fat.

And the changes didn't stop there. I found a new zest for life, sharing this message of juicing and health with the world. In this book, you'll meet some of the people I've helped along the way. And after you complete the challenge (and you will, because I'm going to support you every step of the way!), you too can serve as a beacon of light, a positive influence on everyone whose life you touch. Smoothies are only the beginning on this amazing journey to the best health of your life!

My story goes to show that we really are in this together. So are you ready to get started? Let's do this!

-Drew

PART I: INITIATION

Digestion, Elimination, and Cleansing

What is a Cleanse and Why Would We Want to Do It?

Cleanses seem to be all the rage these days, so much so that they've moved from their previous place, relegated to the back corners of health food stores and alternative health circles, to the mainstream, with many celebrities boasting results from things like the Master Cleanse. But what is a cleanse? And why would anyone want to do one, anyway?

Cleanses can take a few different forms. Usually, they involve restricting certain foods in order to give the digestive system a break so that your body can focus on healing. There are other types of cleanses that involve herbal supplements, but we're going to focus on the food stuff in this book.

So you're probably wondering, what types of foods do you usually eliminate on a cleanse? The foods you want to eliminate are those that are hard to digest or otherwise take a toll on the body. Things like dairy, gluten, and sugar are big offenders here. They can all cause inflammation in the gut, which in turn can cause a broad range of digestive problems and a host of other symptoms, including fatigue, brain fog, aches and pains, skin irritation, etc. Inflammation has even been implicated in serious diseases like cancer. Our goal with a cleanse is to give the body a break from these foods, cool down the inflammation, and let the body work on healing itself so we can experience greater health and vitality.

Health is really just the first step, too. Greater bodily health frees you up to pursue your passions in life and make an impact on the world instead of constantly tending to sicknesses or simply not having the energy or motivation to do anything but the bare minimum.

And cleansing is the first step on this road. As you may recall from the Intro, I experienced a significant change in my digestion after my juice cleanse. By healing the gut, you too will be able to absorb and assimilate more nutrients from your food, which means you'll have fewer cravings for the unhealthy stuff. We generally crave heavy, dense foods because our bodies are searching for nutrients.

The 10-Day Smoothie Challenge can be thought of as a cleanse. We're going to be eliminating all solid foods in favor of fruits, vegetables, herbs, nuts, seeds, and superfoods. Our bodies are going to be stronger and healthier in just ten days!

Digestion and Elimination Primer

In order to get a better grasp on why we're doing this cleanse (you'll find out soon why "why" is so important…hang in there!), let's talk about poop! Seriously, though, it's important to understand digestion and elimination in order to get the most out of this experience. Digestive health is so important to overall health because it doesn't matter as much what you eat as it does what you absorb. If you're not absorbing the vital nutrients in your food, you'll crave more food as your body searches for the vitamins, minerals, macronutrients, and micronutrients that it so desperately needs on a daily basis.

Digestion begins in the mouth. We've heard it before, but it's true. The age-old saying is, "Chew your liquids." Even when drinking juices and smoothies, we need to CHEW. Chewing releases digestive enzymes carried by saliva that mix with food particles and begin the digestive process. Chewing your food will relieve strain on your other digestive organs that only have to work harder when you don't chew enough.

After food is chewed, it passes through the esophagus to the stomach. The stomach secretes hydrochloric acid to further break down food. Did you know that poor chewing habits decrease hydrochloric acid production and that your body produces less and less hydrochloric acid as you age? The rate rapidly declines after age 50; this is why we see so many older adults with vitamin B12 deficiencies, and poor protein and calcium absorption. But these deficiencies (which can cause serious neurological disorders) aren't relegated to senior citizens. B12 deficiencies are quite common in the population at large, regardless of dietary preferences or age (it was previously thought that getting enough B12 was mainly a concern for vegetarians and vegans since B12 is primarily found in animal products). For the sake of your digestion, it's vital to maintain healthy B12 levels. Check out this video (http://fitlife.tv/video/how-to-build-your-hydrochloric-acid) for a pickle recipe that does just that.

In the small intestines, food particles are further broken down and then absorbed into the bloodstream where they can be transported to and used by the rest of the body. Waste products are then pushed through to the large intestines (colon) where any remaining nutrients are absorbed along with excess water, and the waste is turned into stool. Stool is stored in the rectum until it is released in a bowel movement.

And now we come to elimination. I know it's not that popular to talk about bowel movements, but it's an important diagnostic tool to see how your internal organs are functioning. So now for a poop primer! You should be having at least one bowel movement per day, every day, and ideally between one and three. You should never have to strain or push. It should generally be about a foot long and be one long piece. Your poop should smell earthy but not too strong. It should be a dark brown color. Red or black can indicate bleeding somewhere along the digestive tract. Green can indicate that your liver and gallbladder are taxed and are not producing a proper amount of bile salts. Floating poop can indicate that your body is not absorbing fats well (a great reason to do a cleanse and get your digestion working properly again). There generally shouldn't be a lot of wiping, either. Wiping can be a sign that you have a fiber deficiency. Luckily, we're going to be getting lots of healthy fiber in the 10-Day Challenge!

What Ailments Can Cleansing Help?

As we've already covered, many modern ailments can be traced back to inflammation of the gut. Headaches, fatigue, bloating, constipation, gas, brain fog, skin ailments (including acne and eczema), depression, excess weight— even though they may seem disparate, they are often intimately related. Encouraging the body to clean out stored toxins and cool down inflammation will go a long way towards treating these conditions and many others.

Why Smoothies?

Smoothies are a great introduction to a healthy lifestyle. They are super simple to prepare, only require one piece of equipment, and generally taste pretty great. Even kids like them! They're also a great way to reintroduce healthy foods if you've slipped back into old habits and have started overdoing processed foods and sugars.

Also, when you blend your food, your digestive system doesn't have to work as hard. This frees up energy for your body to work on healing all those ailments we listed above!

The Importance of Mindset

Chances are you've tried a lot of things in the past to lose weight and be free of the common ailments and aches and pains that led you to this book in the first place: diets, exercise programs, workshops, retreats, supplements, medications… And you've probably found little success with these regimens or you wouldn't be sitting here, considering a smoothie challenge. Am I right? I'm going to let you in on a secret. This secret is the key to unlocking your greatest potential, not only in the area of health but also in your work, your relationships, and the rest of your life.

Ready to know what this secret is? It's all in your **mindset**. You've probably heard it before: you've got to think positively and visualize what you want. Maybe you thought it was a bunch of baloney, but the truth is that this stuff works! I am living proof of that.

So how can you use the power of your mind to reach your health and fitness goals? Like I always say, if you can go there in your mind, you can go there in your body. The key is education, visualization, and belief. One little trick we're going to use during the next ten days (and hopefully after that, too) is affirmations. We'll talk about those more on Day 1. For now, just know that they're totally easy to do but they provide a payoff. We all need more of those things in our lives, right?

It takes 21 days to form a habit. If you're interested in getting fit for life, this 10-Day Challenge will get you halfway there. Once you realize the power of your momentum, it will be easy to keep going and keep succeeding.

Figure Out Your "Why"

Why do you want to do the 10-Day Smoothie Challenge? Why do you want to lose weight, get healthy, have more energy? Do you want to have more energy to play with your kids or grandkids? Do you want to be able to enjoy the outdoors more and find the joy in moving your body that can only come if you lose weight and have freedom of movement? Do you want to find success in your business or work?

It's vital to get clear on your "why." Without a reason to succeed and push forward, most people fail. It's no different for this 10-Day Challenge. Think of the next ten days as a training ground for the rest of your life. Practice finding your "why" for this challenge and you'll soon find that you can find a "why" for continuing a healthy lifestyle.

Ultimately, it's not about losing weight. Sure, looking good often leads to feeling good, but that's only part of the equation. You're not only getting to your ideal body through this journey, you're getting to your ideal *mind*. Once you reach your goal of your ideal body weight, all you'll need to do is keep your mind clear and focused and you'll never have trouble maintaining your weight again.

Preparing for the 10-Day Challenge: Get Psyched!

What you'll need

All you need for the 10-Day Challenge is a blender and the foods listed in the smoothie recipes you choose to make. That's it! Don't think you need to run out and buy a fancy blender, either (unless you want to, of course!). No need for a Vitamix or Blendtec. Although they do great work, all the smoothies in this book can be made with a regular blender.

Special Tips for Making Smoothies with a Regular Speed Blender:

1. Blend your liquid and greens first! This will eliminate any potential green chunks and unpleasant texture.
2. Blend the smoothie longer. Simple, right? You can add ice at the end to cool it down if the blending warmed up some of the ingredients.
3. Pre-chop your fruits and veggies. This will cut down on the work your blender has to do.
4. A knife will be handy for peeling and chopping fruits and veggies, and a freezer will be great for storing fruits and ice cubes to take your smoothies to the

next level of deliciousness, but I'm assuming those are already in your kitchen.

What's Out:

Meat, dairy (except whey protein isolate), coffee, sugar, grains, all processed foods. No solid foods—put it in your blender!

What's In:

Fruits, vegetables, nuts and nut milks, seeds, superfoods, healthy fats, herbal teas, spring or filtered water.

Fitlife Template for Super Shakes and Smoothies

The following is a general formula for creating super healthy, super delicious smoothies that will keep your energy up and provide all the essential nutrients you need. Not all of your smoothies need to follow this formula, as you'll see in the recipes, but this is a great template to use when you want to get creative and come up with your own combinations while covering all of your nutritional bases.

Keep in mind that not all of the steps below are mandatory. If you don't want a topper, you can leave it out. If you want extra veggies, go for it. If you are trying to keep your calories down, you can manipulate variables like portion sizes and carb and fat content.

STEP 1

Pick a liquid or base:

- Water
- Vegetable Juice
- Almond milk (unsweetened)
- Coconut milk

- Hemp milk (unsweetened)

Less liquid = thick shakes. More liquid = thin shakes. 6-12 oz is a good starting point.

STEP 2

Pick a protein powder:

- Rice protein
- Pea protein
- Hemp protein
- Whey isolate protein (no whey concentrate because it contains lactose)
- Egg white protein

Your powder should be between 15-30g of protein, less than 6g of carbohydrate, less than 2g of sugar, and preferably at least 2g of dietary fiber. Find the protein supplement that you digest well and enjoy the taste of as flavors and consistencies vary widely.

STEP 3

Pick a veggie:

- Dark leafy greens: spinach, Swiss chard, kale
- Pumpkin, sweet potato
- Beets, beet greens
- Cucumber, celery
- Juiced vegetables or powdered greens supplement

Spinach is usually your best bet when you're starting out, as it is virtually flavorless in your shake or smoothie. To remove a lot of the bitterness from dark leafy greens, you can also remove the stems and spines and use only the leaves. Canned organic pumpkin is great, too. It goes well with vanilla. When using beets, try roasting them and removing the skin first. Beets go well with chocolate. If you add celery or cucumber, make sure to adjust the amount of liquid you add.

Add 1-2 fist-sized portions.

STEP 4

Pick a fruit:

- Apples
- Bananas
- Berries
- Cherries
- Dates
- Pineapple
- Mango
- Powdered fruit supplement

Bananas give an excellent consistency, but **one-half** of a banana is a serving size due to its high sugar content.

STEP 5

Pick a healthy fat:

- ½ ripe avocado
- Walnuts
- Flax, hemp, chia seeds
- Cashews
- Almonds
- Almond butter

STEP 6

Pick a topper/extra:

- Coconut flakes
- Cacao nibs or powder
- Cinnamon
- Ice cubes (if using fresh fruit)
- Organifi Green Juice

A little goes a long way. Cinnamon is good with vanilla or pumpkin AND it helps stabilize your blood sugar levels!

So, how about an example? Here's one of my favorites:

- Step 1: unsweetened vanilla almond milk (just enough for it to blend)
- Step 2: 1 scoop of vanilla pea protein powder
- Step 3: 2 kale leaves (just leaves, no leaf spine) & 1 tsp powdered greens supplement
- Step 4: ½ frozen banana
- Step 5: 2 thumbs of walnuts
- Step 6: Top with a few sprinkles of coconut and 5 ice cubes

Let's take a look now at some of the best foods in each category and **why** you would want to choose these superstars over others.

Liquid Bases

Coconut water – aids digestion, settles an upset stomach, and replenishes electrolytes, which makes it perfect to drink post-workout or on hot summer days. It is miraculously compatible with human blood and has been used in the tropics for life-saving blood transfusions.

Nut milks – be sure to buy unsweetened varieties. Or better yet, make your own! Check out this video to learn how to make homemade nut milk with cashews. These creamy beverages are a great alternative to dairy, which can cause problems for a lot of people.

Water – filtered, like reverse osmosis, or spring water is best…but not spring water from a plastic bottle! In addition to the plastic itself being questionable, many companies, including Aquafina and Dasani, have come under scrutiny for actually bottling tap water. Tap water can be loaded with pollutants, pesticides, fluoride, herbicides, estrogen-mimicking hormones, heavy metals, and even pharmaceutical drugs. According to Senator Frank Lautenberg (D-NJ), there are more than 140 chemicals in our water supply that aren't regulated by the EPA. Some of these chemicals include rocket fuel and gasoline. Some brands also add various ingredients to their water to make it "taste better." What most people don't realize, however, is that many of these ingredients are unhealthy or even dangerous, especially for pregnant women. So stick to spring water from a real spring (findaspring.com is a great resource) or invest in a home filtration system that includes three separate stages of filtration: removing sediment, removing chlorine, and a granular carbon filter (this will remove hormones, herbicides, and drugs).

Protein and Healthy Fats

Protein consists of amino acids, which are the building blocks of the body. Every cell depends on protein to maintain, rebuild, and renew itself. When recovering from a workout or injury, protein becomes even more essential.

Fats have gotten a bad rap over the years, but thankfully, that's beginning to change. Fats are vital for healthy skin, good elimination, absorption of fat-soluble vitamins and minerals, and, believe it or not, fat loss! Eating fat doesn't make you fat; excess sugar and processed foods do.

Both protein and fat will keep you full longer and promote satiety (satisfaction) so you're less likely to experience unhealthy cravings. Awesome foods in this category include:

Quality protein powders (hemp, pea, rice, egg white, whey) – an example of a good brand is Sun Warrior. Whey isolate protein powders are also a good option because they **do not** contain lactose (dairy sugars) like their similar counterparts, whey concentrate protein powders. Egg white protein powders are certainly acceptable during this challenge, just make sure you digest it well. Hemp, pea, and rice protein powders are found in any health food store and in many supermarkets. As noted above, experiment to find one you like. They vary a lot in flavor and texture.

Avocados – contain many compounds that reduce inflammation in the body. High oleic acid content helps protect against heart disease. They also promote blood-sugar regulation, which can help ward off insulin spikes that lead to weight gain.

Coconut – coconut has become somewhat of a superstar lately with coconut oil, coconut milk, and coconut water appearing on many a grocer's shelf. There's good reason for this, though. Most of the fat in coconut is made up of medium-chain triglycerides (MCTs). These unique fats go straight to the liver where they are used as a quick energy source. This gives your digestive system a break. They can also be turned into ketone bodies, which have shown promise in treating conditions like epilepsy and Alzheimer's. MCTs rev up your metabolism, helping you burn more calories per day while resting (who doesn't want that, right?). Lauric acid contained in coconut kills yeast, fungus, and bacteria. Coconut also improves blood cholesterol levels.

Pecans – contain oleic acid, which promotes heart health and prevents breast cancer. Of all the tree nuts, pecans are richest in antioxidants. Have been shown to reduce blood pressure. Rich in vitamin E, which provides neurological and cellular protection.

Macadamia nuts – made up primarily of monounsaturated fats, which promote cardiovascular health and weight loss. Contain phosphorus and manganese, which are responsible for bone and teeth mineralization, formation, and repair. Copper content assists in the production of neurotransmitters.

Cashews – copper content promotes energy production. Rich in antioxidants and minerals. Protect skin and hair pigment. Support relaxation and bone health with their magnesium content. Have been shown to prevent gallstones.

Hemp Seeds (hearts) – a complete protein containing all nine essential amino acids (meaning they can't be produced in the body). Provide a balance of essential fatty acids, which are beneficial to brain health, circulation, and blood pressure. Reduce the symptoms of PMS. Are anti-inflammatory. Promote muscle recovery. Treat dry skin and dry hair. Improve organ function and immunity.

Chia Seeds – an ancient superfood prized by the Aztecs and Mayans, chia seeds have recently taken the health world by storm…and with good cause. They are loaded with healthy omega-3 fatty acids, antioxidants, a host of vitamins and minerals, quality protein, and fiber. They promote a feeling of fullness, which can aid in weight loss.

Special note on peanuts – despite the name, peanuts are actually a legume. Because of their porous shell, they are prone to absorbing pesticides, bacteria (remember those peanut butter recalls due to salmonella contamination?), and fungus, including aflatoxin, which is one of the most potent known carcinogens. **Avoid!

Fruits and Veggies

Even the most conservative of health information sources have been telling us all to eat more fruits and vegetables. So there's no excuse here! Even if you don't think you like a lot of foods in this category, use this challenge as an opportunity to expand your palette. I promise you'll find that in no time, you'll be craving healthier foods as a result. Some excellent choices include:

<u>Cucumbers</u> – very high in silica. Silica is great for your skin, nails, and hair. Full of anti-aging compounds. Also very hydrating—one cucumber contains the equivalent of about 3 cups of water!

<u>Kale</u> – nutritional powerhouse rich in vitamins A and C, calcium, antioxidants, and anti-inflammatory compounds. It is especially rich in vitamin K, which has been shown to reduce the risk of some cancers. Per calorie, kale contains more iron than beef.

<u>Spinach</u> – rich in a new category of nutrients known as "glycoglycerolipids," which have recently been shown to protect the lining of the digestive tract from damage, especially damage due to inflammation. Has been shown,

more than other vegetables, to protect against aggressive forms of prostate cancer.

Chard – contains thirteen different polyphenol antioxidants. Anti-inflammatory. Supports the body in detoxing. May help regenerate pancreatic cells.

Celery – protects against inflammation in the digestive tract. Good source of vitamin K, folate, and potassium. Rich in antioxidants. Celery is a very hydrating vegetable.

Parsley – reduces bloating. Inhibits tumor formation, especially in the lungs. Rich in antioxidants and vitamin K. Protects against rheumatoid arthritis.

Apples – their polyphenols have been shown to help regulate blood sugar. The soluble fiber can lower the level of fats in the blood. Consuming apples promotes the growth of beneficial bacteria in the large intestine. Current research indicates that apples may have a positive benefit for a range of conditions, including asthma, cancer, heart disease, macular degeneration, and Alzheimer's. An apple a day really does keep the doctor away!

Lemons – one of the most alkalizing foods on the planet. A great start to your day is a glass of warm water with fresh lemon juice squeezed into it. This wakes up your digestive system and alkalizes your blood. You want your blood to stay more on the alkaline side. If you eat a lot of acid-producing foods (processed foods, meat, dairy, sugar, and gluten), your blood will actually leach minerals from your bones to keep itself alkaline. This is a leading cause of osteoporosis.

Blueberries – contain one of the highest antioxidant levels of any food. Current research suggests that blueberries provide a boost to brain health, specifically in the realm of memory. They are a low glycemic index food, meaning they won't spike your blood sugar. They are also rich in vitamins C and K and manganese.

Strawberries – America's most popular berry. Strawberries are rich in antioxidants and numerous anti-inflammatory compounds. Consumed in modest amounts, they have been shown to effectively reduce certain inflammatory markers in the body such as C-reactive protein. Strawberries are off the charts in terms of their vitamin C content, which helps reduce risk factors for cardiovascular disease.

Pineapple – good source of many vitamins and minerals, including B1 and manganese, which support proper energy production at the cellular level. Super high in vitamin C. Provides immune support and protection against macular degeneration.

Cherries – packed with antioxidants. Reduce the risk of cancer, Alzheimer's, and stroke. Have been shown to reduce belly fat (the most dangerous place to carry excess weight). May help combat insomnia.

Superfoods, Herbs, & Spices

This is where you get to add some zest to your smoothies and literally spice things up! Feel free to use these ingredients liberally—they are called "super" foods for a reason—but a little tends to go a long way. All of the foods in this category contain extraordinary health properties that will make you feel fantastic, prevent disease, and increase your longevity.

Fulvic Acid – one of the byproducts of natural decomposition, fulvic acid is a natural organic electrolyte. Enhancing the availability of nutrients in the body, it helps the body to digest and absorb the vitamins and minerals present in the foods we eat.

Ginseng – a slow-growing perennial plant that traces its roots to ancient Chinese medicine. Known as a natural stimulant, ginseng boosts the immune system, helps to reduce stress levels, and is believed to have properties that are capable of lowering blood sugar levels.

Maca – this root that's related to radishes is sometimes known as "Peruvian ginseng" as it comes from the Andes mountain range. Growing at altitudes above 10,000 feet, this hardy root is an adaptogen, helping cells to resist outside stressors. It is prized for its ability to regulate hormones—both male and female—providing mood stabilization and increased sexual health. It's also great for increasing energy and stamina, especially for athletes. It's most commonly found in powdered form and is readily available online and in health food stores.

MSM – one of my favorite superfoods, MSM does it all! An organic form of sulfur, this compound increases the permeability of cell walls, allowing nutrients to enter more freely and toxins to exit. This speeds up almost every reaction in our bodies, translating to numerous health benefits, including increased joint and bone health, detoxification assistance, skin and hair health, and increased energy.

Mucuna – found worldwide in woodlands of tropical areas, this plant produces pods containing L-dopa, which later converts to dopamine in the brain. Amongst its many health benefits, mucuna has properties believed to help with energy, mood, and libido.

Noni – from small evergreen trees grown in certain regions of Asia and Australia, this fruit is high in phytonutrients, selenium, and vitamin C. Known as an immune system booster, noni has properties believed to help with headaches, migraines, hypertension, and cholesterol levels.

Spirulina – once a food source for the Aztecs and Mayans, these algae are truly remarkable. Rich in protein and a vast array of nutrients, spirulina is basically a daily vitamin in a teaspoon. It is best known for its ability to boost the immune system, but it has a wide range of health uses and benefits.

Chlorella – this micro-algae is a powerful detoxifier that can help rid the body of heavy metals like mercury. It is over 50% protein. It is also rich in chlorophyll, which helps the body process more oxygen, regulate blood pressure, and build and repair tissues. This superfood is most often found in chewable tablet form.

Blue-Green Algae – one of the most nutrient-dense foods on the planet. The great thing about algae is that the nutrients are easily absorbed by the body, which isn't the case with many foods that the body has to work to break down. Like chlorella, it is rich in chlorophyll and has a high antioxidant content. It also consists of over 70% protein!

Cacao (powder or nibs) – one of the most potent antioxidants known to exist. Contains a high amount of magnesium, which promotes relaxation, healthy bones, and regular bowel movements. Cacao keeps your arteries clear, reducing the chance of a heart attack or stroke.

Goji Berry – native to southeastern Europe and Asia, the "wolfberry" has been thought for centuries to prolong youthfulness and life. Rich in vitamin A and antioxidants, goji berry promotes a strong immune system and good vision. Also combats heart disease.

Gotu Kola – a member of the parsley family, this plant has been used for medicinal purposes for centuries in India, China, and Indonesia. Now mostly associated with strong memory function and increased longevity, gotu kola also assists with wound healing and skin problems.

Lucuma – native to the Andean valleys of Peru, this subtropical fruit is rich in nutrients like beta-carotine, iron, zinc, and vitamin B3. Sweet-tasting but low in natural sugars, lucuma does not create blood sugar spikes. Helps with immune system health.

Wheatgrass – prepared from the common wheat plant (though harvested when still short and green), wheatgrass provides chlorophyll, amino acids, minerals, vitamins, and enzymes. One of the world's most ancient foods, wheatgrass helps with alkaline balance, hemoglobin production, and body detoxification.

Turmeric – a root that is commonly ground into a powder and used as a spice in Indian cuisine, especially curries. Turmeric has had value for thousands of years in India, both as food and as medicine, and it has recently been proven to contain high amounts of anti-inflammatory compounds and antioxidants. Turmeric shows promise in treating and preventing a host of Western diseases, including Alzheimer's, cancer, heart disease, arthritis, and depression. It is especially impressive in its tumor-shrinking capabilities.

Vanilla Bean – grown in just a few places around the world, these beans grow on small yellow flowering plants that are part of the orchid family. High in antioxidants, the vanilla bean has properties believed to assist in strengthening the immune system and relaxing muscle tissue. It also makes smoothies taste great!

Ginger – has a long history of use in treating gastrointestinal ailments, especially in traditional Asian medicine. The ginger root is primarily composed of starch with small amounts of protein and fatty acids. Safe to use during pregnancy to reduce nausea and vomiting. Powerful anti-inflammatory that assists in treating arthritis and reducing inflammation in the GI tract. May inhibit the growth of colorectal cancer cells and destroy ovarian cancer cells. Great for boosting immune function—try it out during cold and flu season!

Cinnamon – a popular warming spice that reduces "bad" (LDL) cholesterol and helps regulate blood sugar. Contains essential oils that kill Candida and other fungal overgrowths. The *scent* of cinnamon has even been shown to increase brain function!

Additional Supplements

Want to kick your results up a notch? Try out these supplements in addition to your smoothies:

Apple Cider Vinegar – alkalizes the body and assists in detoxification. Also breaks up excess mucus. Try drinking 1 Tbsp in warm water 2x per day (AM and PM).

Branch Chain Amino Acids – prevents lean tissue loss when in calorie deficit (i.e., while cleansing). Supports fat loss by providing the body with protein's building blocks. Try taking 5g 1-3x daily.

Omega-3 EFA (fish oil) – supports energy levels, cellular function and repair, and brain health. Depending on dietary fat intake, you can take 1200mg EFA 2-4x/day.

Multivitamin – generally, I believe you can achieve all of your vitamin and mineral needs through whole foods, but it's always important to cover all your nutritional bases. When in doubt, supplementation is a great way to ensure that you're meeting your daily needs, especially when doing a cleanse.

Mineral Supplement (Liquid Light) – helps ensure you're meeting all your nutritional needs.

What, When, and How Much to Drink

Optimal digestion does not start with breakfast within 30 minutes upon waking. Start your mornings with two glasses of water or a detoxifying lemon drink; recipe is below. While you're awake, you want to be drinking one 12- to 18-ounce smoothie every 3 hours (ideally 60 ounces every day). Between smoothies, you may drink spring or filtered water, herbal or detox teas. Green tea is ok, even if it contains caffeine. Remember, no solid foods! This is a challenge, after all. ;)

Different types of smoothies are best for different parts of the day. Do your best to rotate your greens and vegetables, achieving a variety of nutrients. You'll want to consume smoothies with higher fruit content earlier in the day or ideally after a workout so that your body can use up that sugar as energy instead of storing it as fat. Smoothies containing high-magnesium foods are great for later in the day to help you relax and wind down for sleep.

IMPORTANT: Prevent macronutrient deficiencies - Include at least 2-3 servings of protein (via powder) and 3 healthy fat options in your smoothies daily.

Lifestyle Factors: Sleep, Stress, Exercise, & Detox

Diet alone will not get you the body or life you desire. It's certainly a great start, but there are other important things to consider as you embark on your health journey. Specifically, we want to look at ways to make this challenge a success for you and as enjoyable a process as possible!

First off, it's essential to get enough sleep every night (that means at least seven hours; eight to nine is ideal), but it's even more important during this challenge because your body will be in a cleansing and repair state. You want to give your body every advantage you can so that you get the results you desire. It's now been scientifically proven that those who sleep less (five hours or less each night) have a higher incidence of overweight and obesity than those who sleep more (more than seven hours each night).

How to get a good night's sleep:

- Stop using electronics (especially televisions, smartphones, and computers) at least an hour before bed. The blue light emanating from the screen signals to your body that it's still light outside and that you should be awake. If you must use these devices at night, use a blue-blocking filter or app or wear blue-blocking glasses.
- Create a bedtime routine. Take a bath (check out this video for a relaxing and detoxifying bath recipe!), read, journal, enjoy conversation with loved ones, reflect on your day. Avoid stressful activities.

- Enjoy a calming pre-bedtime beverage, like chamomile tea with almond milk and cinnamon.
- Create a dark space—blackout curtains, no lights (even lights on clocks and alarms!).

In addition to getting enough sleep every night, this is a good time to experiment with different methods for reducing stress levels. Stress is considered a leading cause of many diseases and it's running rampant in our world today. Stress can come from a variety of causes—everything from an inflammatory diet to strained relationships to work. It's different for everyone and everyone will find success with different stress-reducing methodologies, so it's essential to find one (or more) that you like and that are effective for you. Meditation, yoga, baths, laughter, journaling, talking with supportive friends, and deep breathing are just a few examples. All of these are encouraged during the challenge and beyond. Experiment to find what works for you.

Exercise is also a great way to reduce stress in our daily lives. During the 10-day challenge, however, we are focusing on allowing our body to rest and repair, which means we don't want to push ourselves too hard. Exercise can actually turn into a form of negative stress if our body is trying to recuperate from something or if our system is already taxed to begin with. This can prevent you from losing weight. Because of this, I recommend light yoga or walking as your exercise of choice for the next ten days. Everything in life has a season—take this opportunity to relax and rejuvenate.

Now we come to the subject of detox. I think there are a lot of misconceptions and scary myths out there that we should get cleared up right now. During the next ten days, you're going to be consuming an abundance of healthy food, maybe more than you ever have in your life. Because of this, your body is going to stop focusing on trying to digest the non-food entering your system and instead focus on cleaning house! Over the years, our bodies accumulate toxins from the air we breathe, the water we drink, the food we eat, and the products we put on our skin and use in our homes. These toxins, which are unrecognized by the body, are stored in fat cells. As you begin to release excess weight, these toxins will also be released and allowed to pass through one of the body's elimination pathways: the lungs, the kidneys, the skin, or the colon. These pathways can sometimes get backed up, though, especially when organ function may not be at peak performance levels or if you've had a long history of unhealthy habits. The most common detox symptoms include constipation, diarrhea, dizziness, skin breakouts, headaches, sore throat, achiness, fatigue, and runny nose. They may be a little annoying, but they are a sign that your body is healing. That's a good thing!

There are ways to help your body through this process, though. Saunas and dry skin brushing will help move toxins through your skin. Enemas and colonics will help keep your colon clear and bowel movements regular. Coffee enemas are especially effective and helpful for the liver, which is your body's main detox organ. A detox bath with Epsom salts and essential oils is great for the skin, the lungs and sinuses (by breathing in the steam), and achy joints and muscles. There are many herbal "detox teas" on the market these days as well that provide multi-organ support. Continue to drink lots of clean water and get plenty of rest, and you'll likely find your detox symptoms to be minimal.

Detox Troubleshooting:

- *If you're feeling anxious*…drink passionflower tea, chamomile tea, or incorporate lavender essential oil.
- *If you're feeling hungry*…drink more water, go for a walk, and take some deep breaths. Ask yourself what you're *really* craving right now.
- *If you're experiencing a migraine*…take magnesium, like Natural Vitality's Natural Calm.
- *If you're having trouble sleeping*…try herbal tea with valerian and chamomile.
- *If you need to relax*…try a bath with lavender oil and magnesium flakes or Epsom salts (see video link above).
- *If you're feeling overly lethargic*…try adding 1 tsp sea salt to your smoothies, consume 1 tsp of coconut oil, or experience the amazing benefits of peppermint essential oil in your smoothies or on the back of your neck (2-3 drops).
- *4, 7, 8 Breathing Exercise* … Breathe in through your nose for a count of 4, hold for a count of 7, breathe out your mouth for a count of 8. Repeat at least 5 times.

It's important to listen to your body during the challenge. If you need a nap, take one. If you're thirsty, drink. If you need support, get in touch with our community and we'll help you in any way we can. You are not alone.

Breaking Your Cleanse — coming down

It is important to break your cleanse properly. Your digestive tract has had time to heal, so the worst thing you can do is grab some Chipotle or a three-course meal with your family. You will feel nauseous, disappointed, and bloated.

For the first two days following the Smoothie Challenge, continue with your green smoothie for breakfast. Then for lunch, one of my favorite recommendations is something called a "mono meal." A mono meal is simply when you eat only one type of food and you don't do any kind of food combining. My suggestions are watermelon, peaches, or pears; or roasted or steamed vegetables like carrots, sweet potatoes, or spinach. Avocado is another great choice; or chicken broth as it can be filling and comforting. By dinnertime, you should be ready for a light salad with fresh lemon juice and avocado. Most importantly, listen to your body. You may be craving cooked vegetables, and that is great—simply include these slowly and mindfully. By day three, have a smoothie again for breakfast and a small portion of lean organic meat or plant-based protein with your cooked vegetable or salad at dinner. By day four, you may begin consuming all whole foods with heavier fiber, legumes, quinoa, or beans, but keep it light and healthy. Your body will thank you!

Now that you know everything you could possibly need to know to get started, let's do this!

Prep Days

- **Prepare for the challenge** by cutting back on meat, dairy, sugar, processed foods, and coffee over a period of one to three days prior to Day 1. You will experience fewer detox symptoms this way. Reducing your intake of caffeinated beverages over several days will help eliminate the chance of the infamous "caffeine headache."

- **Go shopping** for the first five days' worth of ingredients. Peruse the recipes towards the end of the book and pick out the ones you plan to make. Make two lists—one for the first five days and one for the last five days and go shopping twice. This way you can have the freshest ingredients on hand. Be sure to stock up on water and herbal or green tea, too.
- **Review your "why."** It's a good idea to keep a journal during the next ten days to record changes, challenges, and insights. You may be surprised at what comes up. Whether on paper or on your computer, record your goals for the challenge and your reasons for participating. You'll want to check in with these every day, so you need to have them written down.
- **Take your "before" pictures.** Take a picture from the front and side and also one of your face. You're likely to see some big changes over the next ten days, so it's important to have a reference point to remember where you came from.
- **Weigh yourself and take your measurements.** You'll only step on the scale once before and once after the ten days to gauge how far you've come. No judgment or berating yourself here! This is just an assessment tool. It's important to point out that we are going for **fat loss** not simply **weight loss**. A lot of crash diets encourage only a loss of water weight, but we are after real, permanent changes. Taking your measurements—your waist, if no others—will be an accurate way to judge whether you're losing fat or water, so measurements are important.
- **Make your entire day of smoothies in the morning.** Refrigerate well. This will make life a bit

easier. You can still have a successful detox if you do not have access to a blender during the day.

- **Join the support community.** It's essential to surround yourself with positive people who will help lift you up when you're having a hard time and will celebrate with you when you experience success. Join our 10-Day Smoothie Challenge community online as hundreds of fellow challengers share their transformations and hold each other accountable (check us out at Fitlifesmoothiechallenge.com). Get motivated and inspired along your journey as participants post their smoothie pictures and results to Instagram using our specific hashtag: #FLChallenge. As if the community and support weren't enough, my team and I also host a monthly prize giveaway! In the first week of each month, we select a winner from our Instagram account...stay on track AND enter to win. Remember, we're in this together! I want to help you every step of the way.

PART II: ACTIVATION

Days 1 – 10

Day 1

The secret of getting ahead is getting started.
- Mark Twain

The hardest part of any journey is often the beginning, but here you are! You have made the decision to start, and you should congratulate yourself for that. Give yourself credit every day for caring enough about your life and your future to embark on this journey. Remember to review your "why" today, to jot down any notes about how you're feeling, and enjoy the delicious smoothies you'll be making. Check in with the community any time you're feeling doubtful, tempted by unhealthy foods, or just want some support.

An Introduction to Affirmations:

Affirmations are positive phrases that you say to yourself to keep you on track. It's a way to infuse positivity into your life from the inside out. We live in a very negative world, and it's easy to let these negative outside influences infiltrate our minds and wreck our mental, spiritual, and even physical health (because you and I both know that the mind and body are inextricably linked). Affirmations work like a shield, keeping your spirits high by deflecting negative outside influences and rewriting negative, habitual thought patterns. Remember, mindset is crucial for success! Practicing affirmations may feel a little funny at first, but it's a great strategy to include in your health plan, especially during a cleanse when you're challenging yourself.

How to "Do" Affirmations:

Affirmations are best said out loud, especially in front of a mirror. They're also great to program into your phone as an alarm at various intervals so that you'll be reminded of your positive intentions throughout the day. When in public, you can read the affirmation to yourself a couple of times and then sit with it silently for a moment, letting its power work through you.

Affirmation for the Day:

I believe in my ability to succeed. My body gets stronger and healthier with each new day.

Stay Connected:

Remember to post a photo of your smoothie today on Instagram with the hashtag #FLChallenge and to visit www.fitlifeSC.com for more details.

Day 2

Problems are not stop signs, they are guidelines.
- Robert H. Schuller

Welcome to Day 2! How are you feeling? Have you noticed any positive changes yet? Did you like the smoothies you had yesterday? Use some of your favorite ingredients from yesterday again today to keep the momentum going, and then try something new. It's ok if you don't like every single recipe. This is about trying new foods and a new way of life. And if you're beginning to experience some detox symptoms, remember that this is your body's way of getting rid of toxins and getting healthier. Try a sauna or a bath. Relax and take deep breaths. Detox doesn't mean you should give up; it means you should keep going!

Affirmation for the Day:

My body is lean, clean, and strong. I love my new healthy lifestyle!

Stay Connected:

Remember to post a photo of your smoothie today on Instagram with the hashtag #FLChallenge and to visit www.fitlifeSC.com for more details.

Day 3

With the new day comes new strength and new thoughts.
- Eleanor Roosevelt

Day 3 is often the time when peoples' willpower begins to waver. Maybe you're starting to notice some detox symptoms. Maybe you've experienced some stress at work or with a loved one. Go back to your "why." Do some journaling. This is a great opportunity to study your habitual patterns and uncover the ways in which you hold yourself back. Don't give up on yourself! Every day is an opportunity to make a new choice about how to live your life.

Affirmation for the Day:

I remain strong in the face of challenges. I am resilient.

Stay Connected:

Remember to post a photo of your smoothie today on Instagram with the hashtag #FLChallenge and to visit www.fitlifeSC.com for more details.

Day 4

The will to win, the desire to succeed, the urge to reach your full potential...
These are the keys that will unlock the door to personal excellence.
- Confucius

What positive changes are you beginning to notice? More energy? Better sleep? Clear skin and clear eyes? Maybe your head feels less foggy and your memory has improved. Maybe your clothes are a little looser. Spend some time in self-reflection today and take stock of the new you. Do you like how you're feeling? If not, change something. The power is all in your hands. Continue reducing stress, getting enough sleep, and trying out some of the detox methods we talked about in the beginning of the book. Take care of your body and your body will take care of you.

Affirmation for the Day:

I have the power to change my destiny. I make positive choices to change my life.

Stay Connected:

Remember to post a photo of your smoothie today on Instagram with the hashtag #FLChallenge and to visit www.fitlifeSC.com for more details.

Day 5

Our greatest weakness lies in giving up.
The most certain way to succeed is always to try just one more time.
- Thomas A. Edison

Symptoms come and symptoms go. Emotions come and emotions go. By now, you may be noticing the transient nature of many of the things we take for granted as "permanent," "irreversible," or "unchangeable." We can change anything we want if we stick with it and don't give up. You can have the life and body of your dreams if you persevere.

Affirmation for the Day:

Perfect health is my destiny and birthright. Perfect health comes easily to me.

Stay Connected:

Remember to post a photo of your smoothie today on Instagram with the hashtag #FLChallenge and to visit www.fitlifeSC.com for more details.

***

You've made it halfway through! I want you to take a moment now to recognize your achievement. Did you have doubts at the beginning that you could make it this far? Well, you're here...but don't stop now. You still have five days left.

Time to go shopping for the final five days of the challenge!

***

Day 6

The starting point of all achievement is desire.
- Napoleon Hill

I want you to go back to the beginning of your notes and again read your "why." Does it still make sense to you? Sometimes, as you begin a process of transformation, your goals and reasoning will change. This is perfectly normal and natural. Are you beginning to think bigger now? Do you expect more from yourself now that you know you can do this? Go with it! Record any new goals and desires you have for your future. You're worth it.

Affirmation for the Day:

I am worth it. I am transformed!

Stay Connected:

Remember to post a photo of your smoothie today on Instagram with the hashtag #FLChallenge and to visit www.fitlifeSC.com for more details.

Day 7

If you're going through hell, keep going.
- Winston Churchill

It's been a week. Congratulations! You're a third of the way to creating a new habit. You're probably getting into a routine now with your smoothies and feeling pretty good about your new healthy lifestyle, and that's fantastic! Remember that it takes time to undo a lifetime of unhealthy habits, though. Don't expect everything to change overnight. There will be times when you are tempted to slip back into old ways. Expect it. Prepare for it. When cravings strike, pause. Take a deep breath. Ask, "What am I really craving right now?" It's usually not food. Is it comfort? Companionship? Activity? Excitement? Seek out new ways to fulfill these needs. Make a list of activities to try the next time you feel compelled to eat for reasons other than hunger. Keep the list with you or hang it on your fridge or cupboard. Preparedness is the key to success!

Affirmation for the Day:

I am prepared. I can handle anything that comes my way.

Stay Connected:

Remember to post a photo of your smoothie today on Instagram with the hashtag #FLChallenge and to visit www.fitlifeSC.com for more details.

Day 8

Change your life today. Don't gamble on the future, act now, without delay.
- Simone de Beauvoir

When was the last time you truly did something for yourself? Selfishness has gotten a bad reputation in our culture, but the truth is that you cannot help anyone else if you yourself are not on top of your game. Oftentimes, people are so concerned with everyone else's needs around them that they neglect themselves into ill health, depression, and resentment. Even if you relate to the archetype of the giver or nurturer, I want you to realize that you've made a powerful choice for **you** by participating in this challenge. You are taking your life in your own hands and gaining control of your health. You do have the power to change…the fact that you've made it to Day 8 proves it!

Affirmation for the Day:

I am focused. I am driven. I take action easily.

Stay Connected:

Remember to post a photo of your smoothie today on Instagram with the hashtag #FLChallenge and to visit www.fitlifeSC.com for more details.

Day 9

 All progress takes place outside the comfort zone.
- Michael John Bobak

Nine days of only smoothies. Pretty impressive, huh? I bet there was a part of you that thought this whole idea was crazy. Maybe you thought it wouldn't work or that you couldn't stick with it. But here you are, doing what you thought was impossible! Progress, growth, challenge—these are all human desires; drives that make life interesting and fulfilling. We're often scared to go there, though. We worry what people will think or whether we can "handle it" or not. But you're here now. Just nine days ago, your comfort zone was totally different. You've stretched yourself already. You've grown and changed. What other amazing things could you do if you just stepped outside your comfort zone a little bit at a time?

Affirmation for the Day:

I am comfortable outside my comfort zone. I welcome growth and change.

Stay Connected:

Remember to post a photo of your smoothie today on Instagram with the hashtag #FLChallenge and to visit www.fitlifeSC.com for more details.

Day 10

What you get by achieving your goals
*is not as important as what you **become** by achieving your goals.*
         - Henry David Thoreau

You've made it to the final day! Finish strong. Reflect on the journey. How are things different for you now? How has your **mind** changed through this ten-day journey? Despite your goals for physical transformation, often the greater changes we experience doing a cleanse like this are in our minds and spirits. Do you feel stronger, more confident, more hopeful? My desire for you is to have everything you dream of. Hopefully this challenge has proved that you really can do anything!

Affirmation for the Day:

I am powerful. I easily maintain my new healthy habits.

Stay Connected:

Remember to post a photo of your smoothie today on Instagram with the hashtag #FLChallenge and to visit www.fitlifeSC.com for more details.

PART III: LEGACY

A Lifetime of Health: Where to Go From Here

What to do once you've finished the 10-Day Smoothie Challenge:

- **Take your "after" pictures.** Just like before, take pictures of your front, side, and face. Compare the two. What differences do you see? You might be so inspired that you become one of our Transformation stories! (Remember to post your photos to Instagram with the hashtag #FLChallenge for a chance to win a blender, juicer, superfoods, and more!) There is nothing that separates you from the testimonials in this book and on our website. Stick with your new healthy lifestyle and you can achieve all the goals you set for yourself.
- **Weigh yourself and take your measurements.** See any improvements here?
- **Reflect on the journey.** What insights have you taken away from this experience? Read back through your journal entries. What themes emerge? What struggles did you overcome?
- **Pass it on.** One of the greatest gifts that health gives us is the ability to be of service to others. Sometimes

this happens without any effort on your part. Others may stop you on the street, wondering where you got that glow. Friends and family may take notice of your transformation and ask you what you're doing differently. Share your secret. Help them succeed. There is a great satisfaction that comes from helping others through the same struggles you've been through—enjoy it and spread the love!

I'm so proud of you for sticking with this journey. It's not easy to change your habits, but you've taken the first step to better health and a better life over the past ten days. If you want to continue making gains in your health and fitness, the foods you've been putting in your smoothies should form the basis of your diet from here on out. That means you should be mainly consuming fruits, vegetables, nuts, seeds, healthy fats, healthy proteins, and superfoods.

Smoothies are a great addition to any healthy lifestyle, so I hope you'll continue to use them in your daily life from here on out. In addition to smoothies, juicing is also something that I am a big fan of as you may remember from the Introduction. Like blended drinks, freshly made juices allow your body to easily absorb nutrients without expending a lot of energy on digestion. If you're interested in learning more about juicing, hop on over to Fitlife.tv and check out my Juice with Drew system.

You may be feeling a little lost now that you've finished the challenge. So I will ask you, what's next? Just as it was important to have a "why" for the challenge, it's essential to figure out a "why" for your life. What drives you? What do you want to create and share with others? What is important to you? What legacy do you want to leave after you're gone? Spend time pondering these questions and work to align your life with the answers you discover.

Everyone needs goals to propel themselves forward. Figure out what you want and go get it! You've already proven to yourself that you can do anything you put your mind to.

I wish you amazing success and health in the future. I look forward to connecting with you on my website and in the Fitlife community. Remember, we're in this together!

PART IV: RESOURCES

Recipes

Spicy Lemon Detox Drink

Mug of filtered hot water
1 Tbsp of apple cider vinegar
Juice from 1 lemon
⅛ tsp of cayenne
1-2 Tbsp of organic pure maple syrup, raw honey, or coconut nectar
Optional: minced ginger instead of cayenne

Greener Mornings

2 cups kale
2 avocados
1 lemon
1 apple
1 scoop Organifi Green Juice (optional)

Strawberry Kale

2 cups strawberries
2 cups kale
2 stalks celery
1 lemon
1 cup coconut water

Anti-Inflammatory Orange Avocado

3 cups coconut water
1 avocado
½ tsp turmeric powder
¼ tsp cinnamon
1 tsp freshly grated ginger
2 cups spinach
1 tsp raw honey
Fresh orange juice (enough to blend)

Blueberry Coconut Water

11 oz chilled coconut water
½ cup ice
¾ cup frozen blueberries
1 tsp lemon or lime juice
1 tsp raw honey
Dash of cayenne

Coconut Lunar Blue Algae Smoothie

1 Tbsp E3 Live blue-green algae
2 cups coconut milk
1 handful of mint

Mango + Coconut Milk + Chia

¾ cup frozen mango
½ cup coconut milk
Blend. Then add and pulse a few times to combine:
1 Tbsp chia seeds
Optional:
Ground nutmeg

Protein powder
2 Tbsp shredded unsweetened coconut

Greena Colada

¾ cup almond or coconut milk
½ banana
Small handful of frozen pineapple chunks
2 large handfuls of spinach or kale
1 spoonful of coconut butter
1 scoop <u>Organifi Green Juice</u> (optional)

Anti-Inflammatory Pain Relief

½ cup coconut flesh
1 cup frozen cherries
5-8 fresh basil leaves
½ cups coconut water (or water)
1 Tbsp chia or hemp seeds
1 scoop <u>Organifi Green Juice</u> (optional)

Double Green

1 handful of fresh kale
1 handful of spinach
1 pear
1 Tbsp raw almond butter
½ Tbsp coconut oil
1 scoop <u>Organifi Green Juice</u> (optional)
⅓ cup unsweetened almond milk

Beet Carrot Apple Detox

1 small red beet
1 sweet apple
1 thin slice of lemon
1 medium peeled and coarsely chopped carrot
A few sprigs of fresh mint
1-inch piece of fresh ginger, peeled (optional)
Water
*This recipe can also be juiced.

Blueberry Brain Booster

1 cup frozen blueberries
½ small banana
½ cup cucumber
1 Tbsp chia seeds
1 cup water

Strawberry Green

1 stalk of celery
1 cup kale
1 cup strawberries
½ lime (peeled)
1 cup coconut water

Dark Chocolate Green

1 mango
1 cup frozen blueberries
3 cups spinach
2 Tbsp cacao powder
8 oz unsweetened almond or cashew milk

Blueberry Protein

1 cup coconut milk
2 scoops Sun Warrior vanilla protein powder
1 Tbsp maca powder
1 cup blueberries

12th Heaven

2 cups almond or nut milk
2 chard leaves
Handful of fresh wheatgrass
Handful of spinach
3 kale leaves
1 apple
2 kiwis
½ pear
½ mango
2 Tbsp spirulina
Little bit of parsley
7 chlorella tabs

California Dreamin'

¼ mango
½ banana
½ avocado
2 handfuls of spinach
Vanilla unsweetened almond milk

Pecan Delight Smoothie

1 Tbsp chia seeds
2 cups coconut milk
1 cup strawberries
Handful of pecans
½ tsp cinnamon

Tasty Toner

1 cup spinach
3 stalks celery
½ cup diced, seeded cucumber
¼ cup fresh flat-leaf parsley
1 small apple, cored
1 Tbsp fresh lime juice
1 Tbsp fresh lemon juice
½ tsp minced fresh ginger
1 tsp lime zest

Raw Green

½ cucumber, seeded
2 cups torn kale leaves, stems removed
2 cups spinach
1 avocado
2 tsp lemon zest
2 Tbsp lemon juice
1 Tbsp raw coconut oil

Gold Star Shake

1 cup almond milk
1 scoop protein powder
1-inch piece of turmeric
½-inch piece of ginger
½ cup fresh papaya

Suns Out Guns Out Shake

1 scoop vanilla Sun Warrior protein powder
1 handful kale
1 cup coconut milk
1 handful strawberries

Cinnamon Swirl Shake

1 Tbsp almond butter
5 macadamia nuts
1 tsp cinnamon
¼ cup coconut milk
1 Tbsp maca powder

Go-Go Fitlife Protein Shake

1 scoop Sun Warrior protein powder
½ apple
1 Tbsp cinnamon
2 Tbsp chia seeds
1 cup almond milk

Rejuv Smoothie

1 cup coconut milk
1 Tbsp cinnamon
1 cup mixed berries
½ ripe banana
2 Tbsp cacao nibs
1 handful of mint

Man of Steel

1 cup coconut milk
1 handful of blueberries
1 Tbsp chia seeds
2 Tbsp almond butter
1 handful of strawberries

The following recipes contain more fruit. We would like to encourage you to have these specific smoothies after your workouts.

Green Detox

2 cups kale
1 cup coconut milk
¼ medium pineapple
1 tsp cinnamon
½ Tbsp honey
Turmeric
1 cup hemp or coconut milk
½ cup frozen pineapple or mango chunks
1 fresh banana
1 Tbsp coconut oil
½ tsp turmeric
½ tsp cinnamon
½ tsp ginger
1 tsp chia seeds
1 tsp maca (optional)

Healthy Chocolate Frosty Love

1 cup unsweetened almond milk
1 frozen banana
1 Tbsp cacao powder
1 tsp vanilla
½ tsp chia seeds
8-10 ice cubes

Hemp Power

1 ½ cups coconut milk
½ cup water or herbal tea
2 Tbsp hemp protein powder
1 Tbsp organic nut butter
½ cup frozen strawberries
1 banana
1 tsp chia seeds
1 tsp cinnamon
1 tsp spirulina
1-2 ice cubes (optional)

Banana-Berry Green

½ ripe avocado
1 frozen banana
1 cup fresh or frozen blueberries and strawberries
2 handfuls of fresh spinach
1 cup unsweetened vanilla almond milk
1 Tbsp ground flaxseeds (optional)

Spirulina Smoothie

1 banana
1 cup blueberries
1 cup spinach
1 apple
2 cups kale
2 tsp spirulina
1 Tbsp chia seeds
1 cup coconut milk
1 scoop Organifi Green Juice (optional)

Sweet, Creamy Green

1 frozen banana
1 orange
1 avocado
4 cups chard leaves, stems removed
2 cups cold water

Coconut Kale

1 frozen banana
4 cups chopped kale, stems removed
2 Tbsp ground flax
½ cup coconut milk

Beginner Blueberry Kale Smoothie

1 large ripe banana
1 cup frozen blueberries
2-4 kale leaves
1 Tbsp chia seeds or maca powder
1 scoop protein powder
1 cup pure water

Vegan Muscle Builder

½ cup strawberries
¼ mango
½ orange
½ cup green grapes
½ banana
½ cup oats
Ground flaxseed
1 cup green tea
2 cups kale
2 cups almond milk

Minty Chocolate Shake

1 frozen banana
1 handful of cacao nibs
1-2 cups mint
2-3 cups coconut milk
2 handfuls of spinach
1 cup kale
Ice

Smoothie-Tootie

1 ½ cups coconut milk
1 tsp honey
2 tsp ground flaxseeds
2 cups spinach
3 cups kale
1 ½ cups pineapple chunks
1 frozen banana

PMS Rescue

6 oz coconut milk
1 Tbsp cacao powder
1 banana
½ cup strawberries
1 peeled kiwi
3 Tbsp lemon juice

Berry Best

2 cups water
1 cup mixed berries
1 mango
1 cup spinach

Raspberry Ripple

2 cups water
1 cup raspberries
1 banana
1 cup bok choy (pak choi)

Tropical Detox

2 frozen bananas
1 cup fresh or frozen mango
1 cup fresh cilantro
1-2 cups coconut water or water

Perfect Morning

1 frozen banana
1 cup almond milk
2 handfuls spinach leaves
¼ cup walnuts
¼ cup oats
Sprinkle of cinnamon

Anti-Inflammatory Pineapple Ginger

2 cups ripe pineapple
1 cup ripe mango
3-inch piece of ginger, peeled
½ cup celery
1 cup coconut water
1 tsp fresh vanilla

Tropical Kale

3 cups kale
1 frozen banana
½ cup frozen strawberries
¼ cup frozen pineapple
½ cup coconut milk
½ cup spinach
2 Tbsp honey
Ice cubes (optional)

Citrus Pineapple for Weight Loss

2 frozen bananas
2 cups frozen pineapple
1 cup fresh orange juice
Juice of 1 lime
½-inch piece of ginger, peeled
½ tsp nutmeg
2 tsp turmeric
1 cup coconut milk

Pineapple Spinach

½ banana
1 cup fresh pineapple
2 big handfuls of spinach
1 cup water
1 cup ice

Coconut Banana

2 frozen bananas
1 cup coconut milk
1 tsp coconut oil
½ tsp vanilla extract
1 Tbsp chia seeds
2 Tbsp almond butter
1 apple or pear

Simple Green

1 cup kale or collard greens
1 Granny Smith apple
1 banana
½ cup loosely packed parsley

Amazing Green

½ cup water
2 Tbsp flaxseeds
2 clementines, peeled
1 banana
2 cups spinach
½ cup frozen pineapple chunks

Strawberry/Orange

1 banana
1 handful of parsley
1 orange, peeled
½ cup strawberries or strawberry pulp from juicing
¼ to ½ cup fresh juice, water, or coconut/almond milk

Skin Cleanser

1 avocado
2 cups frozen mango
1 cup fresh orange juice
½ cup water
Handful of mint

Minty Lime Detox

1 ½ frozen bananas
Half a lime, peeled
1 orange, juiced
1 handful of mint
½ cup coconut water or water
1 handful of greens (optional)

Thank You

Well, congratulations, you made it! Thank you for believing in yourself enough to go through this challenge. I always say, it is the small steps that lead to big changes in our lives. The past ten days have indeed been hard, but worth it. How good you feel now is just the beginning of taking your transformation to the next level. I'd love to update you on future projects and challenges that I create with my team in San Diego to assist you on your continued path of wellness. So please make sure you subscribe to our email list at www.fitlife.tv.

Also, if you find it in your heart to help me spread this mission of self-transformation to ten million people by leaving a brief review on Amazon, I would greatly appreciate it.

Warm Regards,

Drew Canole

Freebies from Fitlife

Check Out More Products and Services From The Fitlife Team!

Name	URL
Greens Powder	http://bit.ly/1tAqs1v
Juice with Drew	http://bit.ly/1EiMaMo
5 Day Detox	http://bit.ly/1x6uaBu
Workout	http://bit.ly/1okNBWM
Meal Guidance	http://bit.ly/1s55UdM
Coaching	http://bit.ly/1tcHGhV
Membership	http://bit.ly/1okNSJl

About the Author

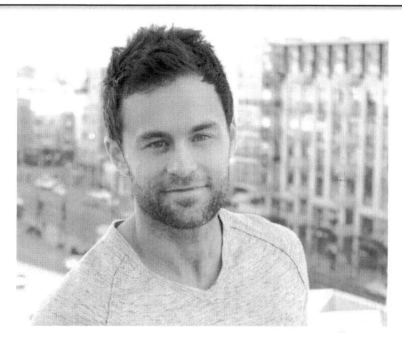

Drew Canole is a nutrition and transformation specialist, well known as a national spokesperson for the benefits of juicing and smoothies for health and vitality. He is the founder of Fitlife.tv where he shares "Educational, Inspirational, and Entertaining" videos and articles about health, fitness, healing, and longevity.

Drew Canole's transformation clients include celebrities, entrepreneurs, CEO's, authors, and personal development gurus.

The success of his first book, *Juicing Recipes*, vaulted him to national attention as a first-time author and has garnered media and television attention in the form of book deals, TV talk show hosting, and national endorsements from some of the leading national companies focused on health, wellness, and athletics.

Canole believes everyone has greatness inside them but they need the right fuel to bring it out.

Made in the USA
Lexington, KY
25 November 2014